21 EXERCISES FOR
THE 21ST CENTURY

21 EXERCISES FOR THE 21ST CENTURY

◆

A SELF-HELP PROGRAM OF SIMPLE ISOINTEGRAL EXERCISES FOR PAIN-FREE LIVING

Greensufi

iUniverse, Inc.
New York Lincoln Shanghai

21 EXERCISES FOR THE 21ST CENTURY
A SELF-HELP PROGRAM OF SIMPLE ISOINTEGRAL EXERCISES FOR PAIN-FREE LIVING

iUniverse, Inc.

For information address:
iUniverse
2021 Pine Lake Road, Suite 100
Lincoln, NE 68512
www.iuniverse.com

ISBN: 0-595-30397-8

Printed in the United States of America

Dedicated to my loving sons,
Haleem and Kabir

CONTENTS

ACKNOWLEDGEMENT

I am indebted to Ari Burack for his timely assistance in collaborating with me in writing and editing the book. In addition, he drew all the exercises with attention and focus.

PREFACE

One night while sleeping, I turned over to my other side and noticed that the third finger on my left hand was twisted. I could not manage to straighten it. Instinctively I used the other hand to do it.

In the morning, I felt fine. Being in my mid-sixties, it was an awakening that perhaps arthritis was knocking at the door of my hands. I developed an exercise for the hands that not only prevented the continuation of this sudden experience, but also made me quite aware of other possibilities.

Having sustained a hip injury in my early teenage years while playing soccer, I developed a limp as a result. This meant that the body had to be treated with greater awareness.

As a child I traveled with my father south of Delhi, in India, where we met fakirs, mendicants, holy men, and people from a mysterious world then unknown to me. This was my father's way to atone for the loss of his oldest son. The sensations that I felt in my body while there never really left my memory. It was as if I had been thrust into another world and then suddenly pulled back.

Having traveled and lived in the United States in the late 1950s and 1960s, and later on in Europe, the ideas and experiences I encountered connecting the mind to the body began to crystallize within me. For further exploration, my travels led me to Asia. There I became deeply involved in the world of esoterica. The world of vibrations. The "micro-world" within our bodies, and also its ongoing connection with the "macro-world." How this relationship can be sensed became incorporated in my lifestyle.

We have a tendency to address pain (psychosomatic) through different ways. Mostly through pills. We are also addicted to suffering. There is an alternative that we can and should investigate.

The electromagnetic currents going from the body to the brain and back can provide a clue, and can also bring a great deal of relief to our system. Before any kind of pain caused by arthritis, lower back pain, carpal tunnel syndrome, knee joint pain, and even stress, can develop further, we must learn to pay attention to our body. To its breathing, rhythm, and flow. Why don't we?

These simple and doable exercises have been developed for the purpose of the "entrainment" of our highly sophisticated system, and the activation of the neurons found not only in our brains, but throughout our bodies. If I can do them, so can you. I started doing each one for myself, and found them to be quite effective. I then began giving them to friends, both younger and older, with surprisingly good response. It was suggested to me that I provide access to them on a website. They can now be viewed, in live motion, at www.yoga4health.org. Alive and at work.

May these exercises help and benefit all those who are interested in the body as a sacred source of who we are.

A neuronal network with unlimited possibilities, linked to the Cosmos.

Greensufi

INTRODUCTION

We are living in intense and volatile times. Our lifestyles demand that we move, think, make decisions, plan, and perform our tasks at an ever-increasing pace. All the while, less and less attention is being paid to our bodies. The natural flow of life-force, for which are bodies are admirably equipped, is no longer a part of our imagination.

Living more, as it were, in our heads, we become disconnected with the workings of our vital self. This kind of "disembodied consciousness" has allowed our energies to become scattered and unmanageable, and is the root of much of our pain and suffering. We move through our lives as if we consider ourselves to be separate from the natural and solar world in which we are embedded. And yet, where else are we?

This disconnectedness manifests in the body in many different ways. The various organs, including the heart, are being asked to work faster, and breathing has become labored and constrained, leading to a lack of energy in the hands, feet, arms, back, and muscles in general. The blood flow has become constricted. The lymphatic fluid, which is primarily responsible for the development of the immune system, is not circulating properly.

Further, when we are not mindful of the sensations coming from our bodies, we can multiply the problems caused by common conditions such as lower back pain, arthritis, carpal tunnel syndrome, sleep disorders, and stress.

Now your body is certainly not a carcass, simply connected to your head. It is a powerful vehicle for your health, well-being, and wakefulness. You have before you a tremendous opportunity to familiarize yourself with it.

In the ancient Yogic and Tibetan Buddhist understanding of the human organism, the physical body is merely the outer layer covering a series of increasingly subtle layers. *Inside* the physical body lies what is known as the "electrical body," which is connected to the intricate neuronal and lymphatic networks that run through the entirety of the system. This electrical body is vital for a healthy and energized state of being, but remains undeveloped in most people.

Taking the time to become more attentive to the sensations being emitted from and within your body goes hand in hand with learning to recognize and acknowledge the existence of an electrical body. As you grow older and slow down, you become more aware of your feelings, which in turn can help you perceive signals from the electrical/lymphatic system.

The awakening or enlivening of the neuronal networks within your body, through your increased attention and through certain practices, leads you to tap into what is known in Tibetan Buddhism as *fohat* or "fire-mist." As the electrical body matures within you, you become more able to entrain your system to detect any kind of discomfort, anytime. Focus and manipulation of your electrical circuitry becomes useful as well as desirable in order to prevent and avoid pain.

The following simple exercises, created specifically to aid in this development, will help you to heal yourself on an ongoing, daily basis, and will prevent you from having to live in pain—naturally and organically.

EXERCISES

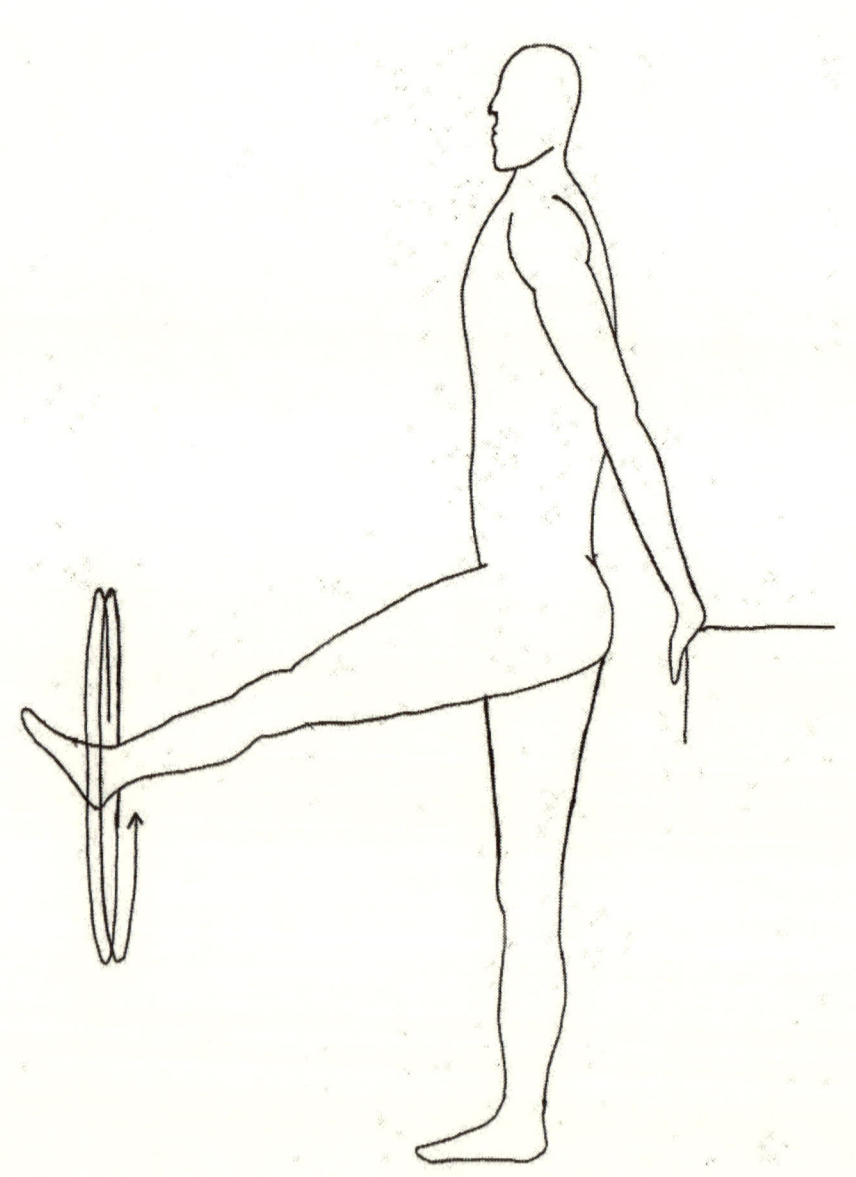

1.
REDUCTION AND PREVENTION OF LOWER BACK PAIN

Standing straight, lift one leg straight ahead, while bracing yourself on a strong surface with the hand on the same side as the lifted leg. Make a circle with your foot, moving your leg around in a direction toward the outside of your body (clockwise if turning your right leg, counter-clockwise if turning your left leg). Make one hundred revolutions for each leg.

Try to get into a slow, relaxed rhythm to help your lower back loosen up. Closing your eyes may help you feel more closely how each part of your leg, hip, and lower back is connected and moving together to help you accomplish this exercise. You will begin to feel your body warming up as you move through the exercise. You may begin to feel that this part of your body is becoming more unified, and this will help you, not only with the exercise, but after, when you are walking, standing, or sitting down. If you have been sitting in one place for a long time (such as at a desk at work), take the time to notice *how* you are sitting. Are you balanced or out of balance? Are you putting pressure on one side of your body? Are you hunched over? If you are noticing the signs of pressure on your lower back, take a break for a few minutes and try this exercise.

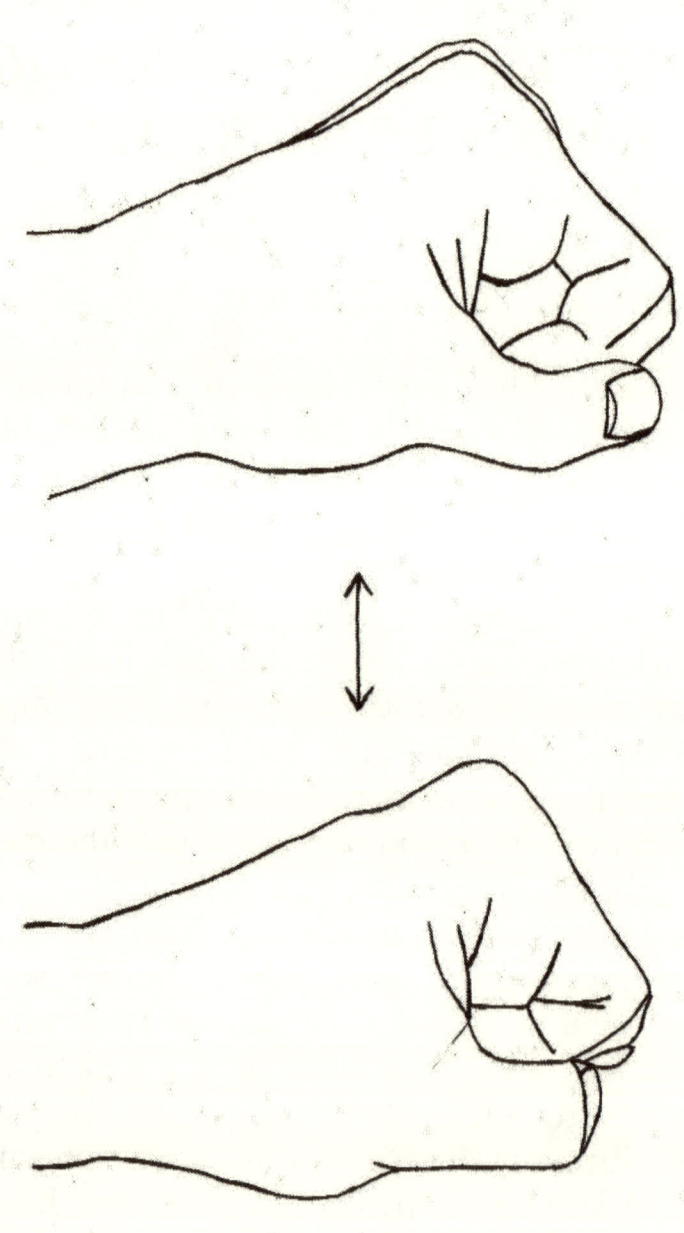

2.
PREVENTION AND EASING OF ARTHRITIS IN THE HAND

Make a semi-closed fist with your hands, wrapping your thumb around the outside of your fingers. Now close your fists tightly, and then release back to the semi-closed position, keeping your thumb on the outside of your fingers. Repeat one hundred times to exercise the muscles of your fingers and hand.

Feel your hands getting warm. Observe your breathing. You can move your breath in a slow, relaxing rhythm with the movement of your hands. When finished, stop and observe the feeling of energy in your hands. Keeping this in mind, you may begin to see how you are using your hands throughout your day: at work, resting, moving from place to place, etc. Does the way you use your hands increase the tension in them to a degree greater than necessary? Doing this exercise can help you observe this, and you can make small but important adjustments.

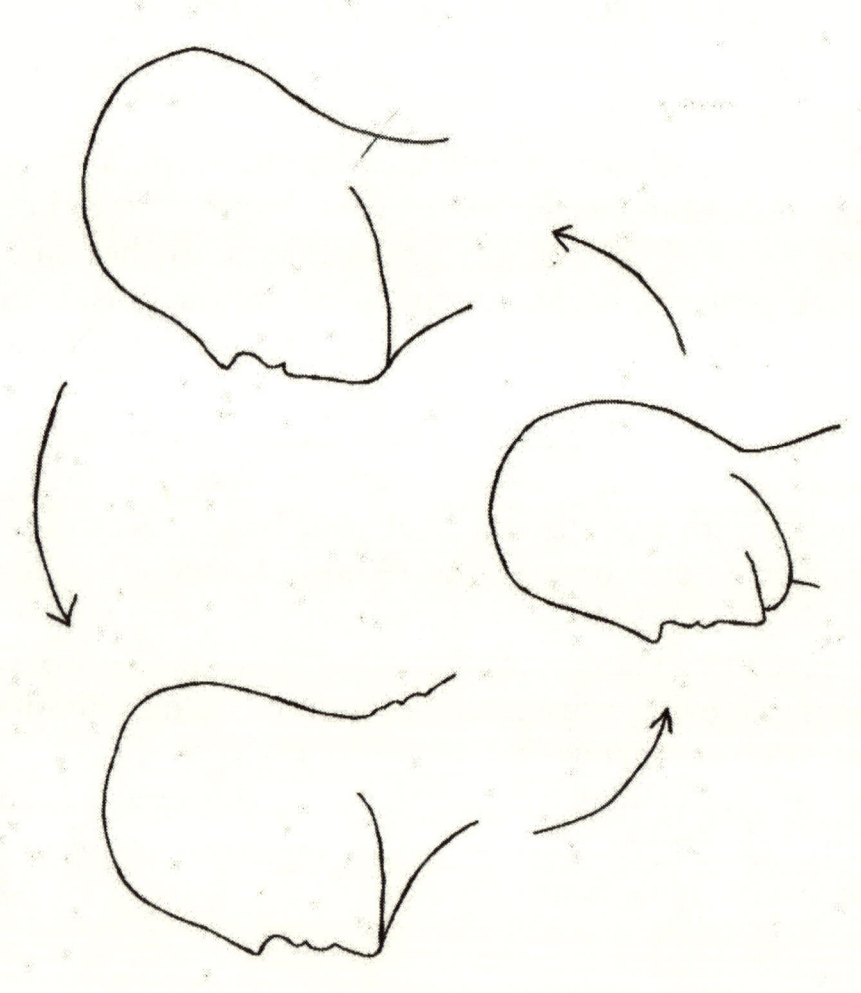

3.
RELAXATION OF THE NECK AND REDUCTION OF NECK PAIN

Facing forward with your neck relaxed, make a forward-directed circular motion with your neck. This should allow your chin to sweep up, forward, then down in front of the top of your chest, and around again and again in a relaxed and rhythmic motion. Repeat one hundred times to loosen up the muscles of your neck and your upper back.

Move purposefully but gently. The neck can be delicate. Breathing is important. Breathe *into* and *through* your neck. Feel the warmth of energy moving from the base of your neck up through your head, rhythmically releasing tension more and more, deeper and deeper, with every circle you make. You may begin to notice this energy pathway in operation even after you complete this exercise, as you will be more relaxed and thus more observant. Feel how you are holding your neck and shoulders. You can begin to bring this observation into the rest of your day, especially when sitting at a desk at work, when concentrating, or in situations that normally cause stress. All of these tensions can accumulate throughout the day and are often stored in the neck and shoulders. This exercise can help to regularly release tension and soothe this part of the body.

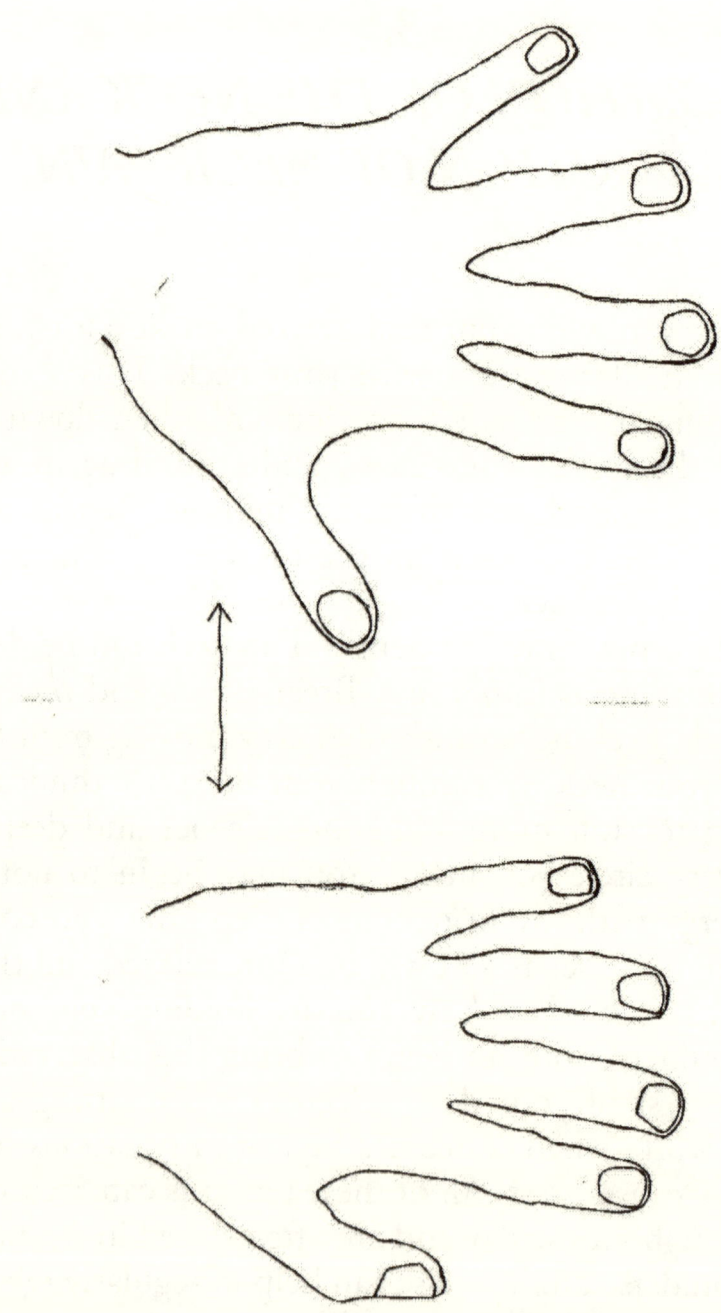

4.
CTS 1: PREVENTION AND EASING OF CARPAL TUNNEL SYNDROME (CTS)

Holding your hands straight out with your fingers relaxed, push out and extend your fingers as far as they can go, and then let them fall back again to a relaxed position. Repeat one hundred times. This exercise helps conditions such as carpal tunnel syndrome, and should be used frequently.

Feel the energy inside your body moving from your wrists up through the tips of your fingers. The warmth helps relax the muscles and joints of your hands and fingers. Take time from work to pause for a few minutes to do this exercise. As with the other exercises, there is no need to move quickly–doing this exercise just to get to one hundred can be counter-productive, or at least not as effective. It is better to take your time and do this exercise slowly and consciously, with purpose. This very intention will increase your overall relaxation and healing capacity.

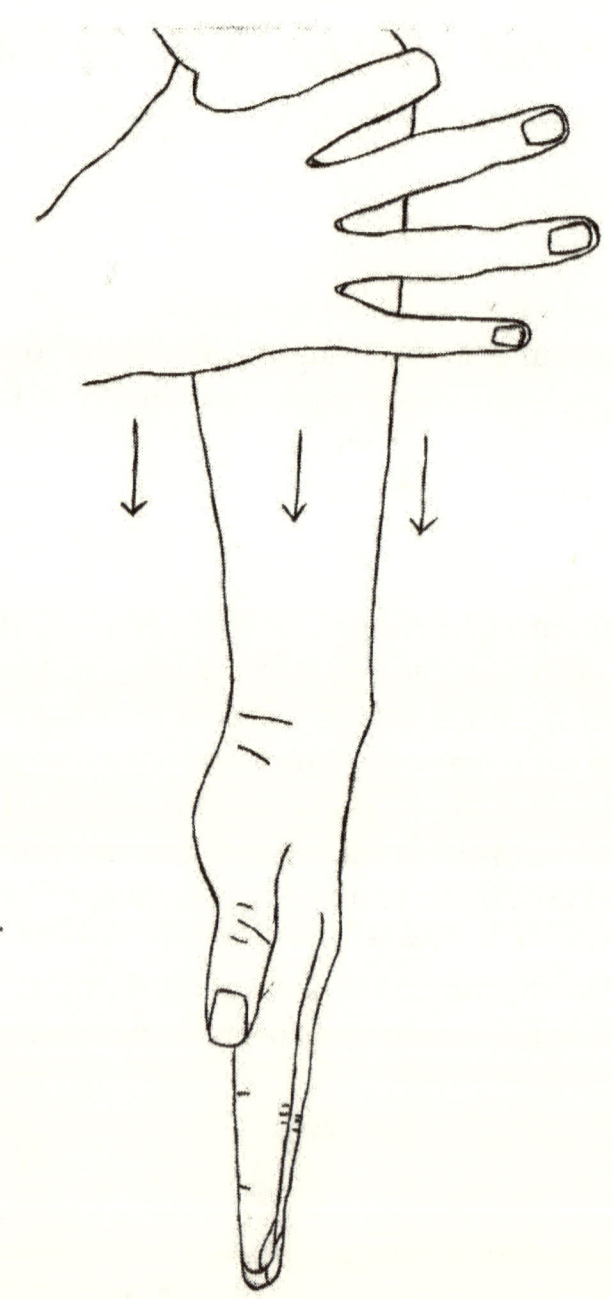

5.
CTS 2: STIMULATION OF THE LYMPHATIC FLUID (HELPS FURTHER ALLEVIATION OF THE SYMPTOMS OF CTS)

Holding one of your arms out in front of you, grasp it at the beginning of the forearm just above the elbow, with the thumb and forefinger of your opposite hand. Then, grasping firmly, slide your thumb and forefinger slowly down the entire length of your arm, past your wrist, and over your hand all the way to the tips of your fingers. Repeat one hundred times for each arm. Use massage oil to facilitate the movement.

The movement and friction of the fingers on your arms creates warmth, a buzzing of energetic activity with the increased blood flow in your arms, in this case moving from the top of your forearm down to your fingertips. Your arms and hands begin to feel more unified and relaxed.

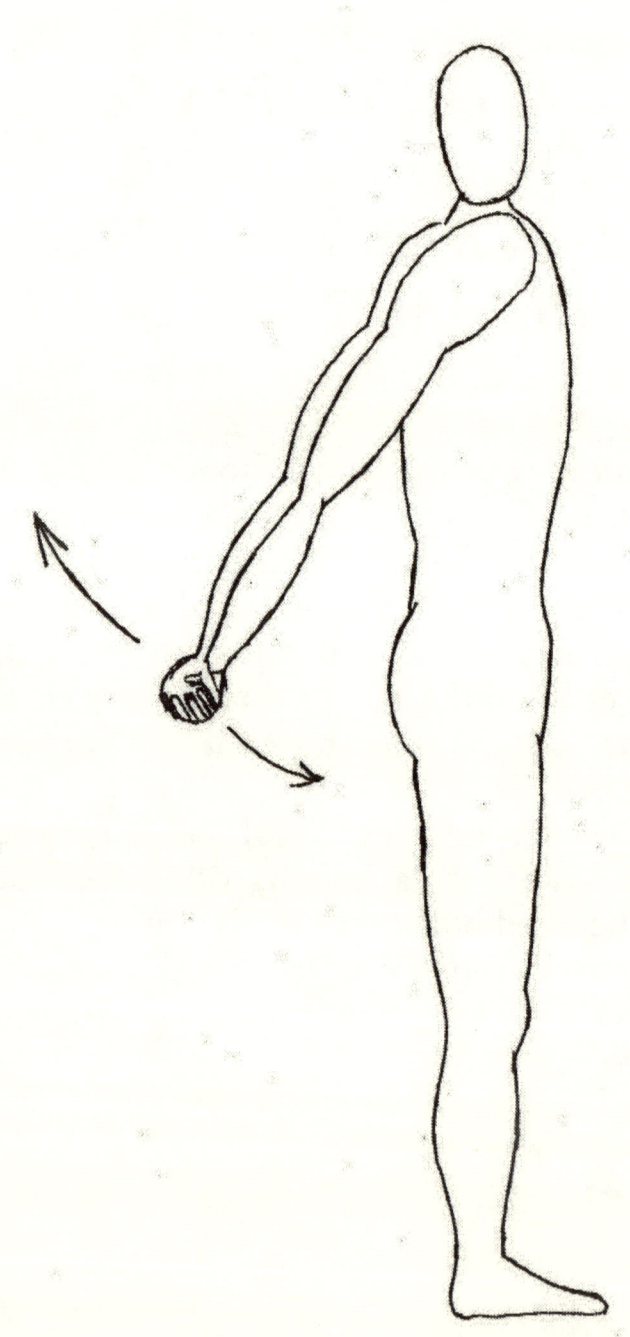

6.
WAKING UP THE NEURONS IN THE BODY

While standing straight, clasp your hands behind your back. With your arms straight and fingers intertwined, rock your arms toward and away from your buttocks. This back-and-forth movement of your shoulders and arms realigns the upper spine, and helps to reconnect the mind-body axis. Repeat one hundred times.

Feel the sensation of warmth being created along the whole length of your spine. Your body feels more awake, more energetic and active, from the base of your spine all the way up to your head. This exercise also helps you focus on your breath, which you can begin to move in rhythm with your arms. This will help you slow down and relax as you simultaneously become more awake and active. Your torso is becoming more unified with your head, and your mind is becoming relaxed and focused, and more able to direct your body in a harmonious way.

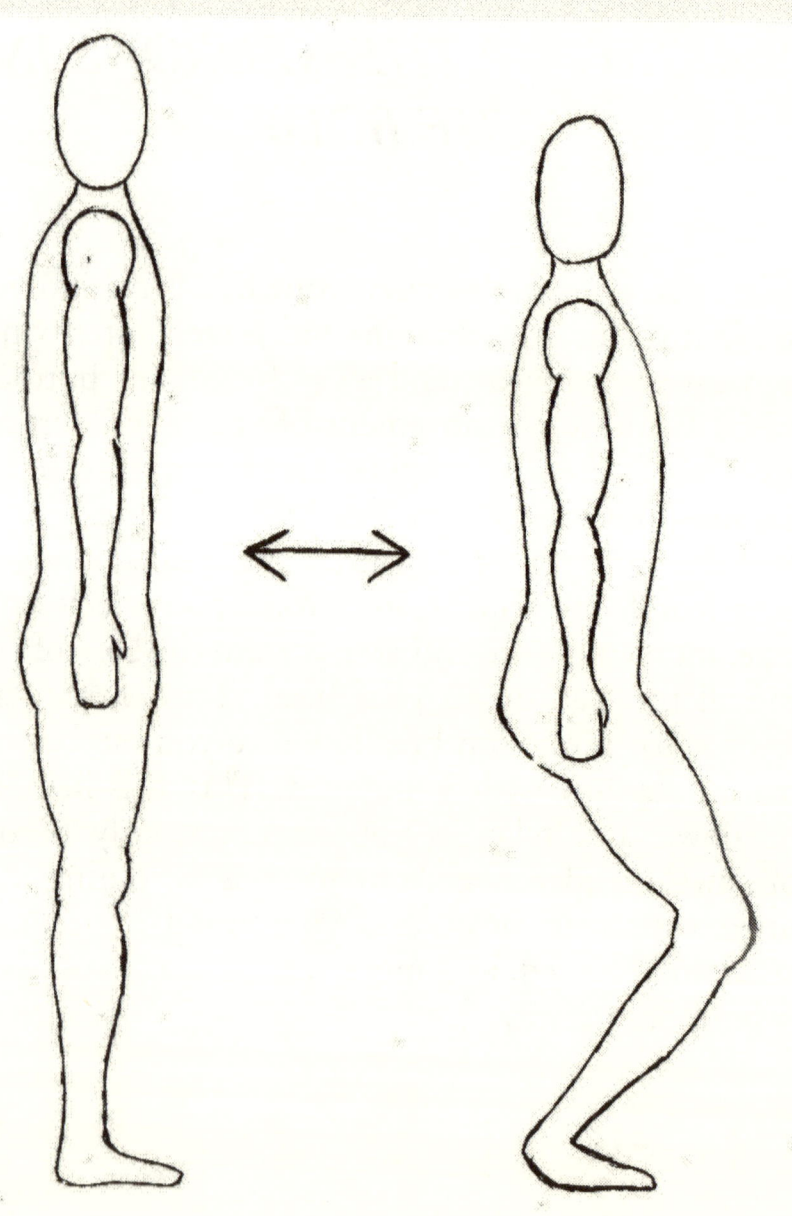

7.
RELAXATION OF THE LOWER TORSO AND UPPER THIGH

Standing straight with your arms hanging at your sides, bend your knees low and then rise up again, keeping your upper torso and head straight. The meeting of the torso and the lower part of the body helps generate more unified electrical activity in the system. Balancing the energies on a daily basis is the key to prevention of back pain. Repeat one hundred times.

This exercise integrates the energies of the lower body with the energies of the upper body. You can begin to breathe in tune with the movement very easily, moving slowly and relaxing the body even more deeply. You may begin to observe the connections between your knees, thighs and back, and how closely they work together when you walk, sit down and stand up, or pick up heavy objects. These observations may seem very obvious, but how many of us pay attention to them regularly, and use this information to make our movements easier and more harmonious? Through this exercise, we can become more aware of these things.

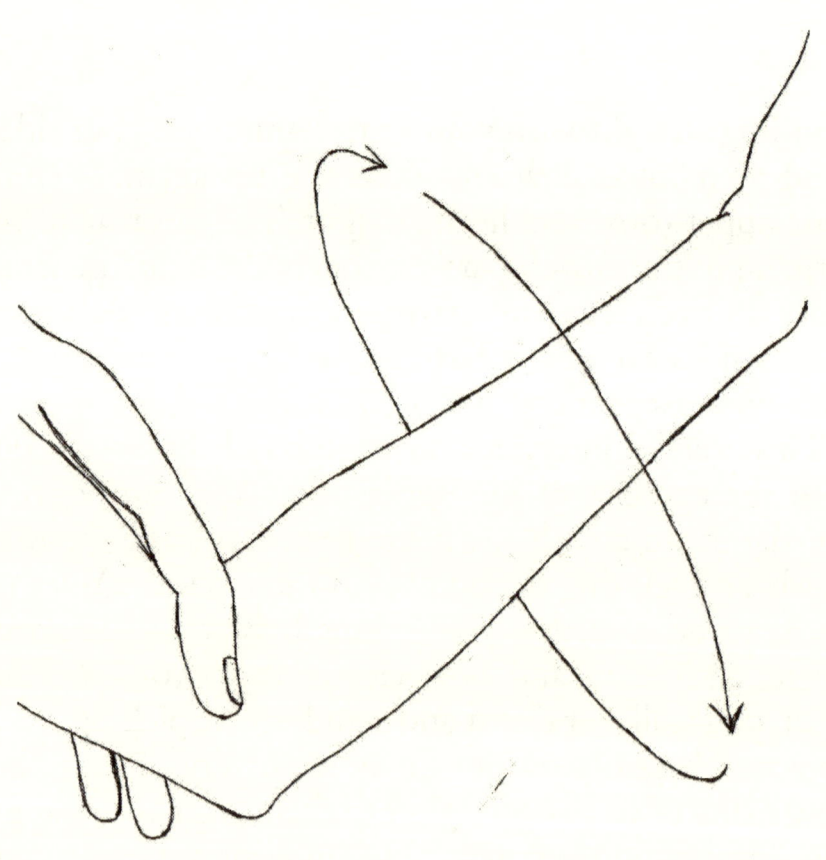

8.
CTS 3: CARPAL TUNNEL SYN-DROME REDUCTION AND PRE-VENTION

Holding one arm out straight in front of you, lightly grasp your arm between the thumb and forefinger of the opposite hand, just above the elbow joint. Swing your forearm and hand around in a circular motion (clockwise for your right arm, counter-clockwise for your left arm), keeping your upper arm straight and stable. If you are working at a computer for a long time, and using your wrists and elbows frequently, it is suggested that you take a few minutes off every two hours and engage in this exercise. Repeat one hundred times for each arm.

This carpal tunnel exercise focuses not only on the hands, but also on the elbows, incorporating the whole of the upper arm in the movement. In addition to relieving tension in more than just your fingers, hands and wrists, as the other carpal tunnel exercises do, this exercise allows you to feel your hands, wrists and forearms in a more unified way, coursing with the energy that allows us to accomplish our daily tasks. Coupled with a few of the other hand exercises, this exercise will provide a more complete regimen for your hands and arms, which can become so intensely taxed throughout the work day.

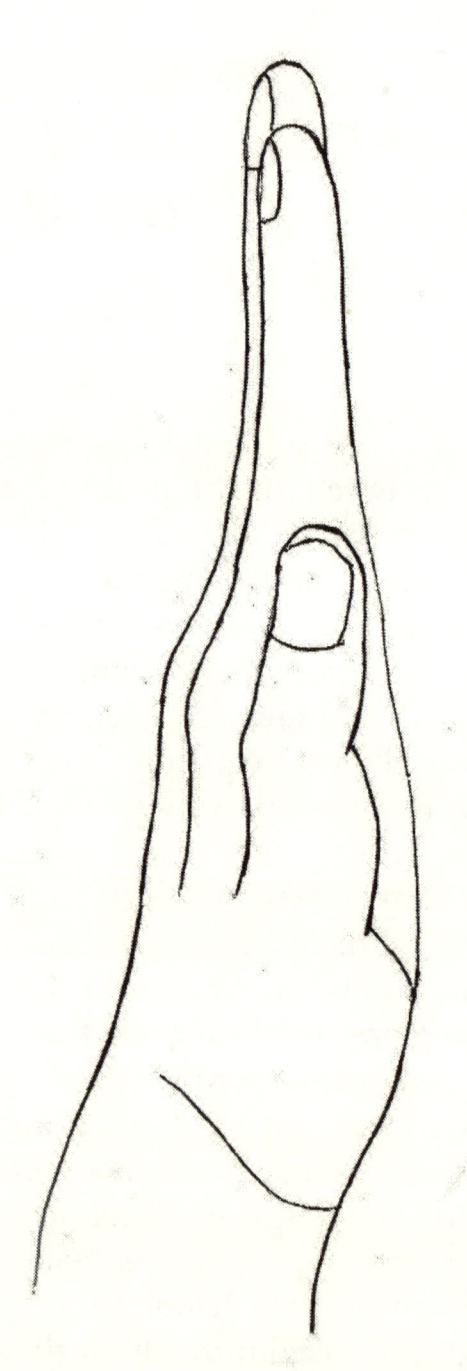

9.
CTS 4: ADDITIONAL EXERCISE FOR CARPAL TUNNEL SYNDROME REDUCTION AND PREVENTION

Holding your hand out in front of your body, begin with your palm facing away from you. Moving your wrist in a circular or spiral motion, curl your hand down and around, ending with your hand again facing away, and repeat, with a slow, natural, flowing movement. Repeat one hundred times for each hand.

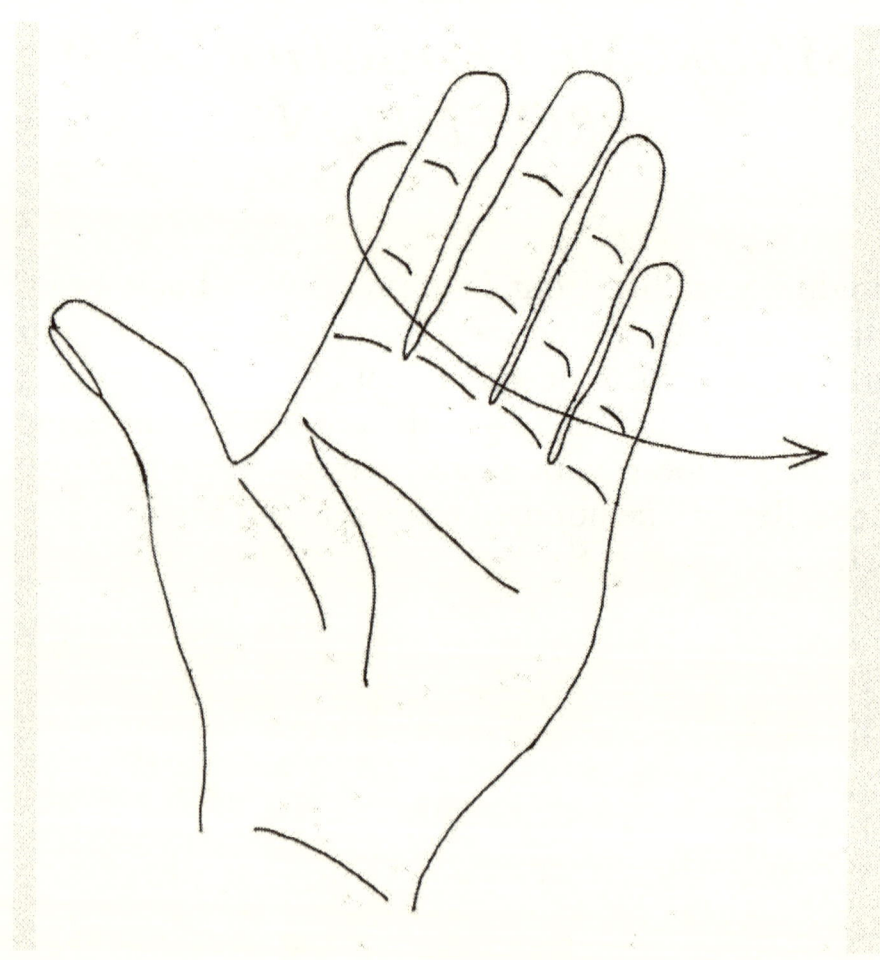

This exercise, in combination with any of the other hand exercises, can be highly useful for regulating normal hand and wrist movement. It increases flexibility in the wrist and hand as well as helping to expel built-up tensions in the hand. In connection with your breath and awareness, it also helps to relax the mind.

In a highly stressful environment, if you are hunched over a computer screen and using your hands and fingers frequently, your lymphatic flow becomes constrained. As a result, greater tension is built up throughout the entirety of your arms and hands. This exercise helps release the lymph, leading to better flow and a relaxed state.

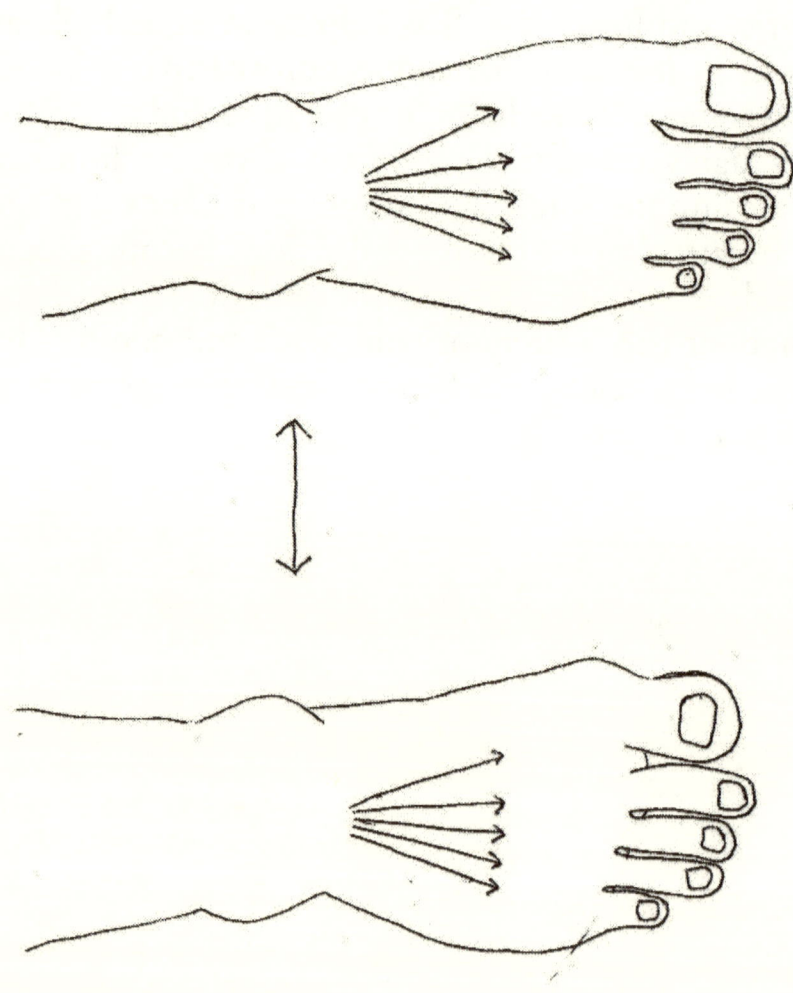

10.
ISOINTEGRAL METHOD OF INDUCING AND AIDING SLEEP

Not being able to relax the mind, and struggling with reducing tension in the body, makes falling asleep more difficult. Slowing down and relaxing your energy, reducing brain wave activity, and re-aligning the mind-body axis leads the practitioner to settle into sleep more easily. While lying down in bed before sleep, locate a point at the front of your ankle joint (facing forward toward the toes). From this point, where the muscles and nerves of the foot begin, flex and release that area, which should raise and lower your foot and toes slightly. Repeat one hundred times for each foot.

This simple, very subtle exercise creates a wave of healing and relaxing energy that moves straight up from each foot to your head. Your mind becomes very relaxed, your body releases tension, your breath becomes calmer and more stable, and sleep comes more quickly and naturally.

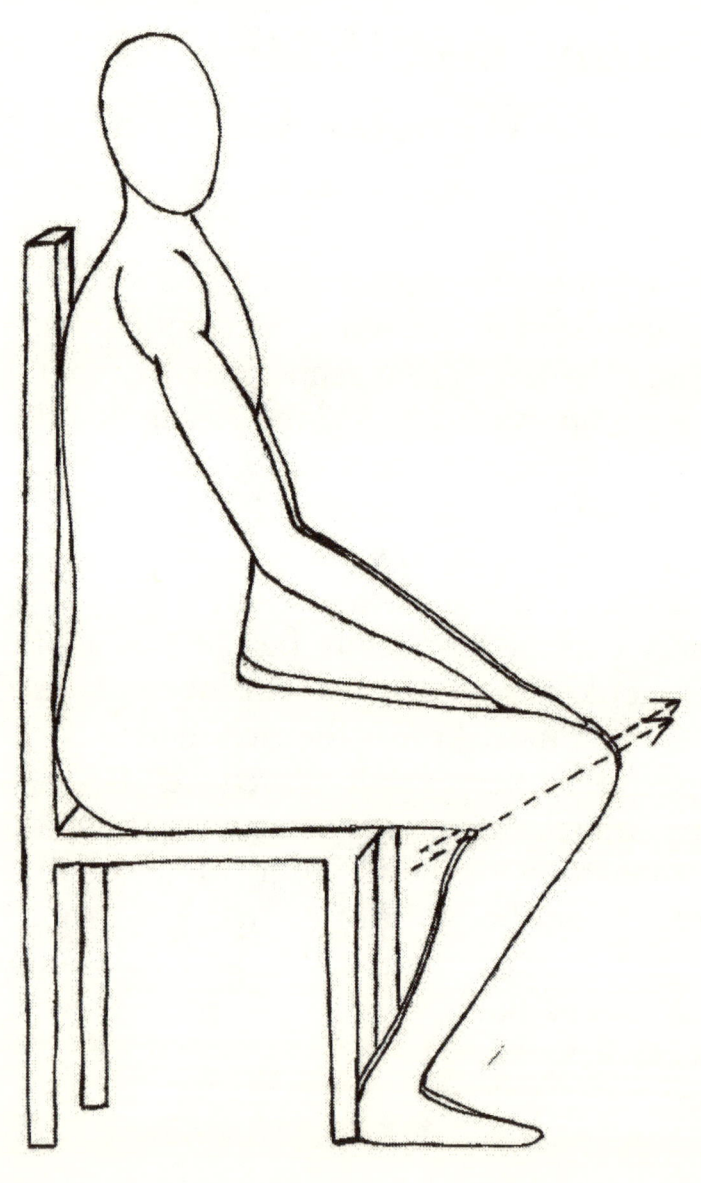

11.
PREVENTION AND REDUCTION
OF KNEE JOINT PAIN

In a seated position with your feet on the ground, locate a point directly behind your knee joint. Repeatedly flex and release from this point, as if an invisible line of force were moving from this point through to your kneecap. Keep your feet on the floor. Your legs need not move, but you may feel the back of your thighs and calves flexing and releasing with this movement. Repeat one hundred times. You can exercise both knees at the same time.

When performing this exercise, you may notice energy and warmth beginning to concentrate in your knee joint. This exercise both relaxes and strengthens the knee in a subtle way. The simplest exercises, done in a positive and open state of mind, can create surprising changes.

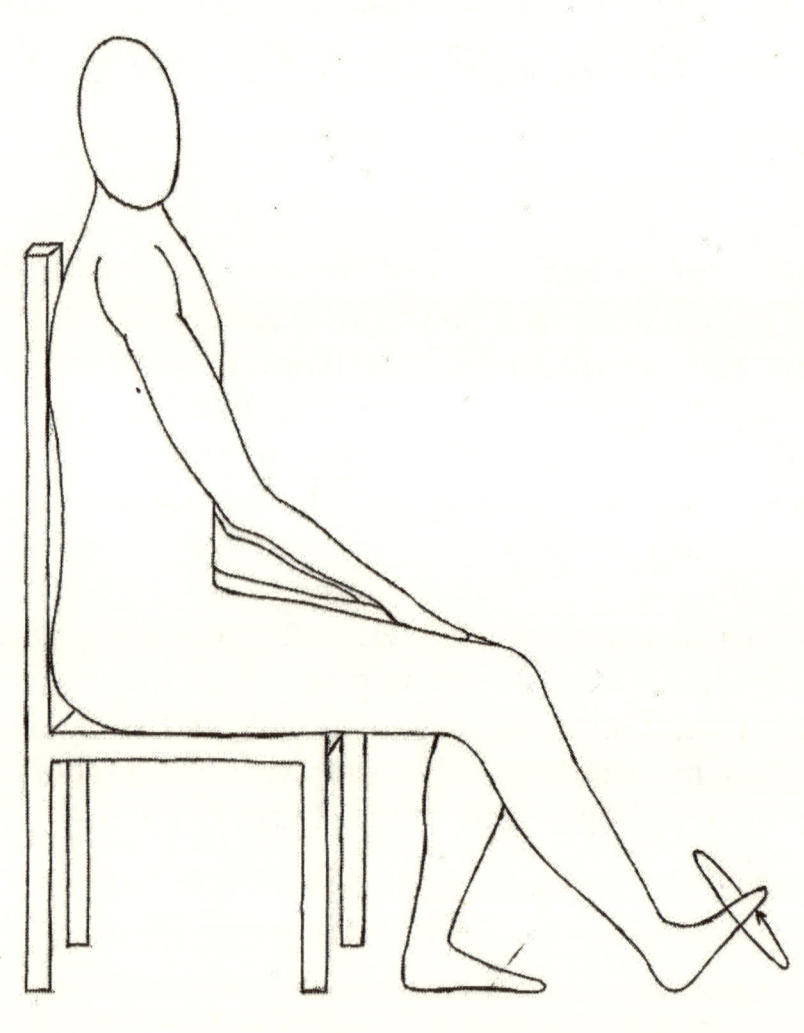

12.
STIMULATION OF THE LYMPHATIC SYSTEM FOR RELAXATION

This exercise can be done in a seated position with your feet on the floor, or while lying on your back (before sleep). While your heels remain on the ground or the bed, rotate your ankle so that your toes move in a circular motion towards the outside of each foot. Repeat one hundred times.

The tension that can build up in the body and mind throughout the day is dispersed through this simple exercise. Since much of the time our minds can become preoccupied with various thoughts, worries, hopes, and fears, this exercise redirects the attention of our mind and body to our feet, to what grounds us with the Earth, the natural world around us. While doing this exercise, feel the spiraling, healing energy being created in your feet as it moves upward through your legs, your back, your stomach, your heart, and up through your head. You may begin to notice your breathing, as it too becomes more relaxed and grounded.

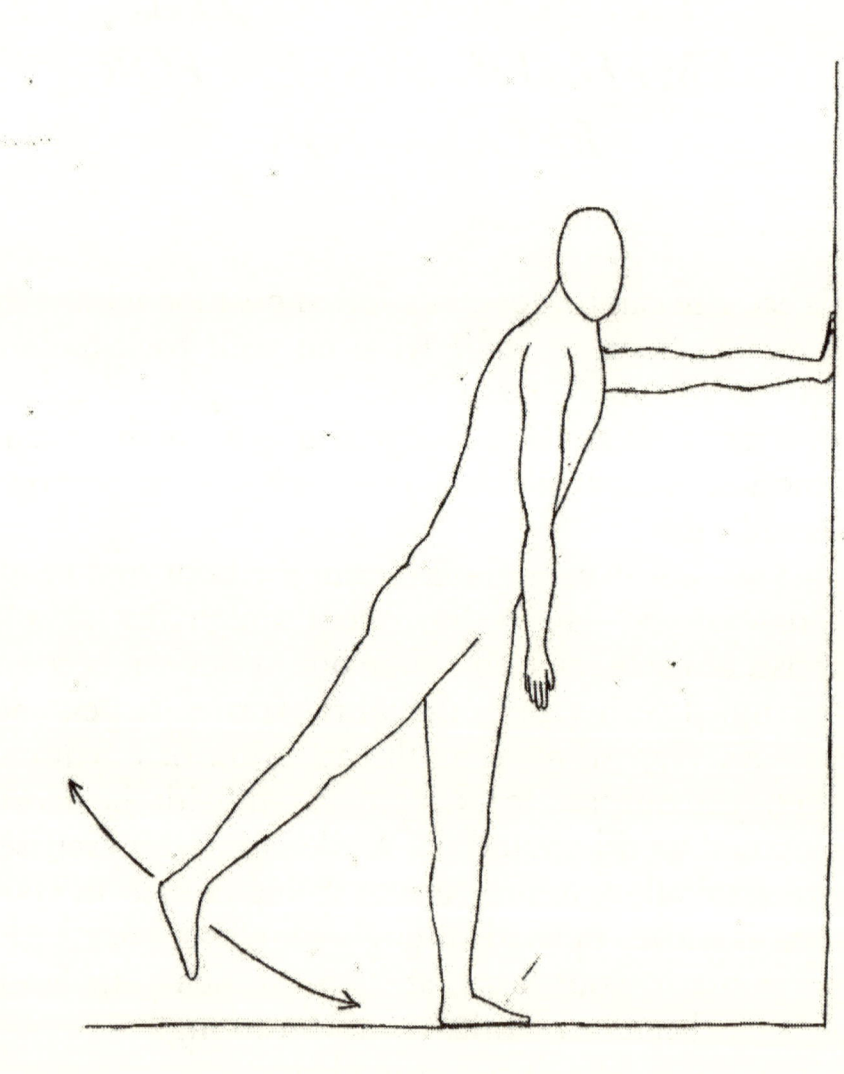

13.
TREATMENT OF LOWER BACK PAIN AND STRENGTHENING OF THE LOWER BACK

Standing straight, close your eyes and, with your arm straight, place your left hand onto the wall in front of you. Raise your right leg behind you, fairly high, and bring it down again, without touching the floor with your foot. Repeat this leg movement up and down slowly, one hundred times. Now place your right hand onto the wall and repeat the same motion with your left leg. If this exercise feels difficult, begin with a few repetitions, and then you can slowly work your way up to repeating it one hundred times for each leg. After this exercise, another exercise is useful in relaxing your back after this first stretch. In the same position, simply bend at the knee and raise and lower your lower leg behind you, and repeat several times for each leg. These two exercises are also recommended in combination with the front-facing lower back exercise (REDUCTION AND PREVENTION OF LOWER BACK PAIN).

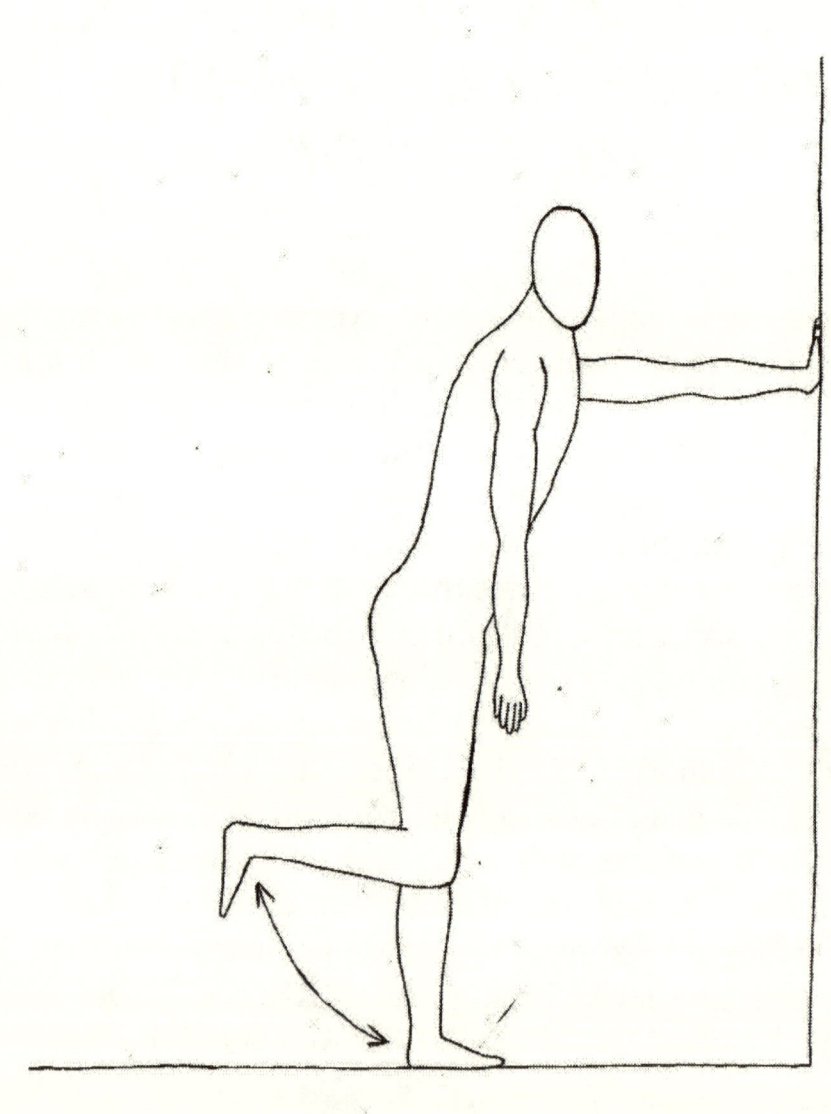

In doing this exercise, it is important to feel your lower body as a single unit. In conjunction with your breathing, you can scan your entire lower body, from your feet, up the length of your legs, to your hips and up your spine. You begin to sense how each of these parts is connected and moving in cooperation with each other. As you repeat this exercise regularly, your lower back becomes stronger and more flexible. You can start to train yourself to feel your legs and back moving together in healthy balance, both during the exercise and afterward, as you stand, walk, and sit. When you move in harmony, tension and strain are diminished, and after a time, are removed entirely.

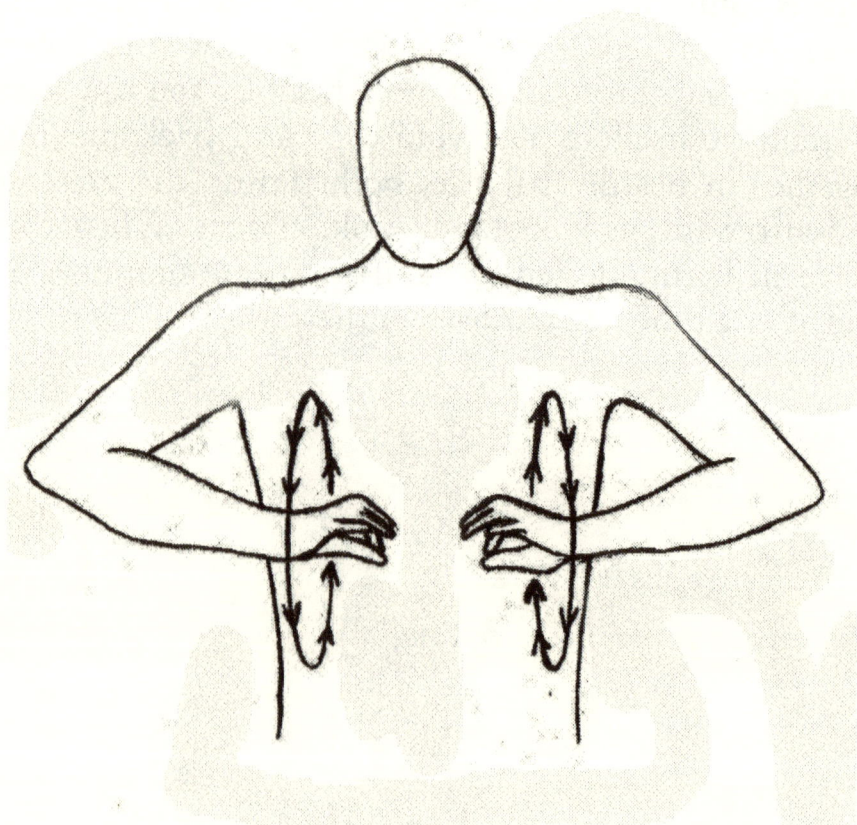

14.
RELAXATION OF TENSION IN THE UPPER TORSO, SHOULDERS, AND ARMS

If you are standing with bent shoulders, as most of us do, there is tension collected in the upper portion of your body. One must learn to release it on a daily basis. Bring your arms and hands parallel to your chest, a few inches from your heart, until the hands are almost touching. Allow the thumb and forefinger of each hand to touch each other, forming a closed position, known as a "mudra." This connection establishes an energy circuit. With your eyes closed, using your elbow as a fulcrum, rotate your arms in a circular fashion away from your body, slowly and rhythmically. Repeat this exercise one hundred times.

While keeping your back straight, sense the release of tension. This exercise generates nerve and muscle activity, and can also be used for arthritis and carpal tunnel syndrome.

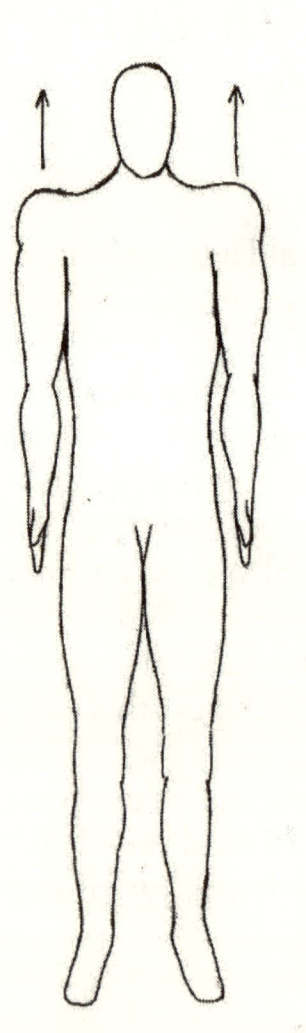
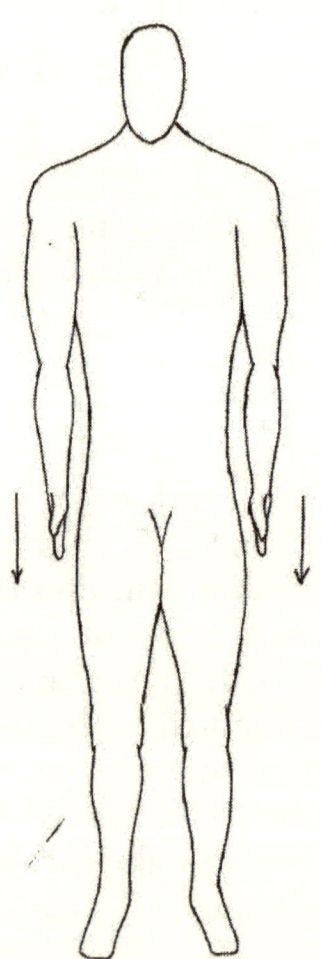

15.
TORSO RELAXATION EXERCISE AND CLEARING THE MIND

Stand straight, close your eyes, and allow your hands to rest at your sides. Push downward gently (not violently) with your hands, allowing your torso to release. This is a gentle, rhythmic thrusting motion. As you push downward, shake your entire arm out, all the way to your hands, along with the upper part of your torso, as if you are shaking off water after a shower. In this case, you are actually shaking off the tension in the body.

Feel the movement of your breath begin to synchronize with the movement of your arms and torso. As the exercise goes on, you begin to sense a clearing of the mind in a way that leads to mind-body integration. Repeating one hundred times is recommended.

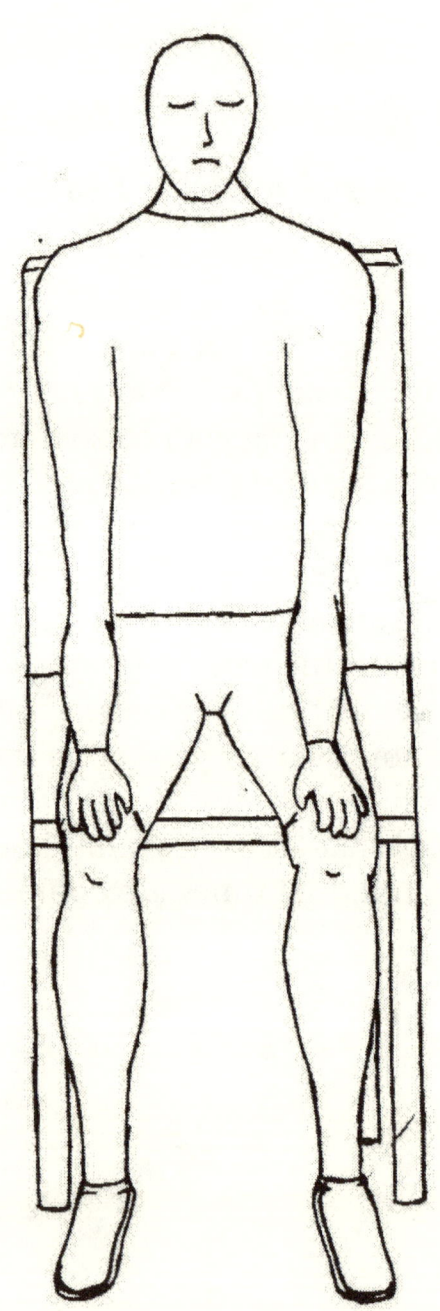

16.
BREATHING EXERCISE FOR STRESS REDUCTION

Sitting in a relaxed and comfortable position, allow yourself to begin to focus more closely on your breathing. Inhale vigorously (but not violently) three times in close succession, until your lungs are completely filled. You can count to three in your mind as you do this. Now hold your breath for a count of four. After holding your breath, exhale vigorously three times until the lungs are empty, and begin the exercise again. We recommend that before this exercise is undertaken, you have cleansed out your system (i.e., evacuated the bowels).

It is not only breathing in and out, as the exercise describes, but also, it is paying attention to your breathing process. Initially, repeating the exercise seven times is recommended, especially for those who are involved with a yoga practice.

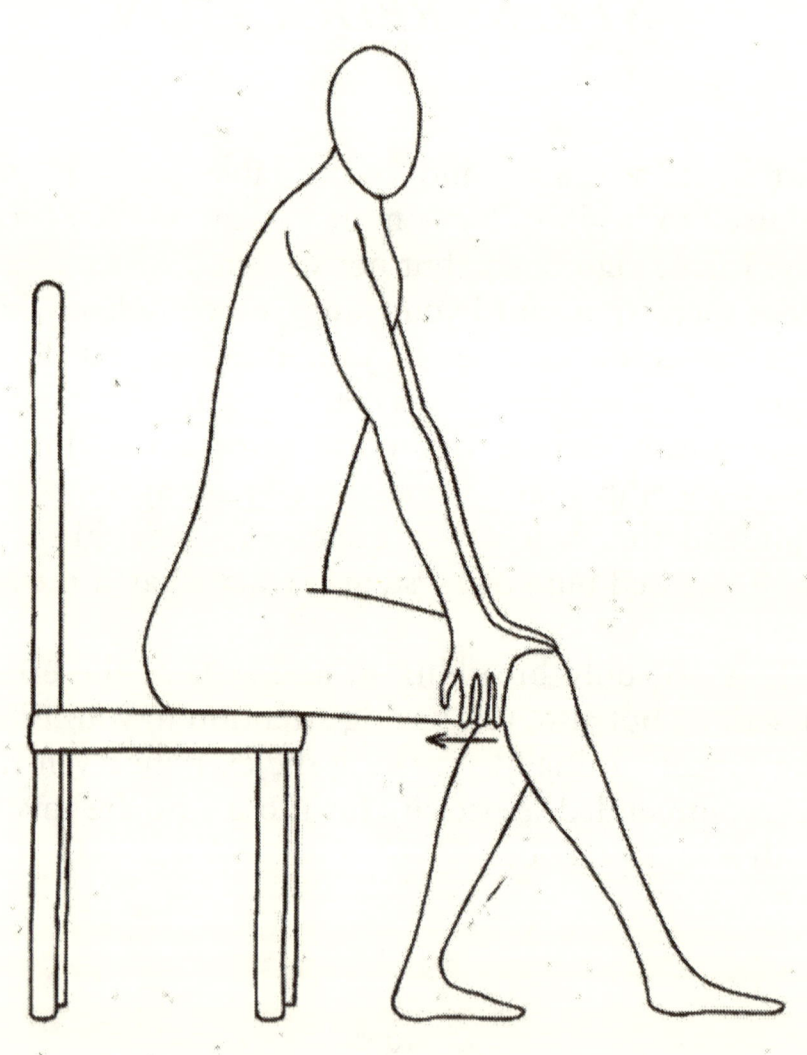

17.
PREVENTION OF STIFFNESS IN THE KNEE JOINT AND RELAXATION OF THE KNEE

The two tendons that begin near the back of the knee and continue up the thigh have a tendency to stiffen from walking, running, and sitting in a certain position, making it difficult to walk without pain.

Sitting in a comfortable posture in a chair with your feet on the floor, place one foot slightly forward, so it is not directly below your knee. Cupping one hand, pour a little massage oil into the palm. Mix it into the other hand. Place the fingers of both hands on these two strong, cord-like tendons at the back of the knee, and your thumbs at a point just above your kneecap. Gently massage with your fingers, from the point where these tendons begin, upward just a few inches along the beginning of your thigh. Move your fingers back to the point where you began and repeat, massaging in a slow, rhythmic fashion until you feel the tendons soften and release tension. Repeat for the opposite knee.

You should begin to feel the whole knee begin to relax, and this sensation of relaxation will move down the leg, all the way to the feet. It is a sensation of cooling and relaxing energy filling the knee and then moving down the leg, as neuronal activity is being stimulated in these areas.

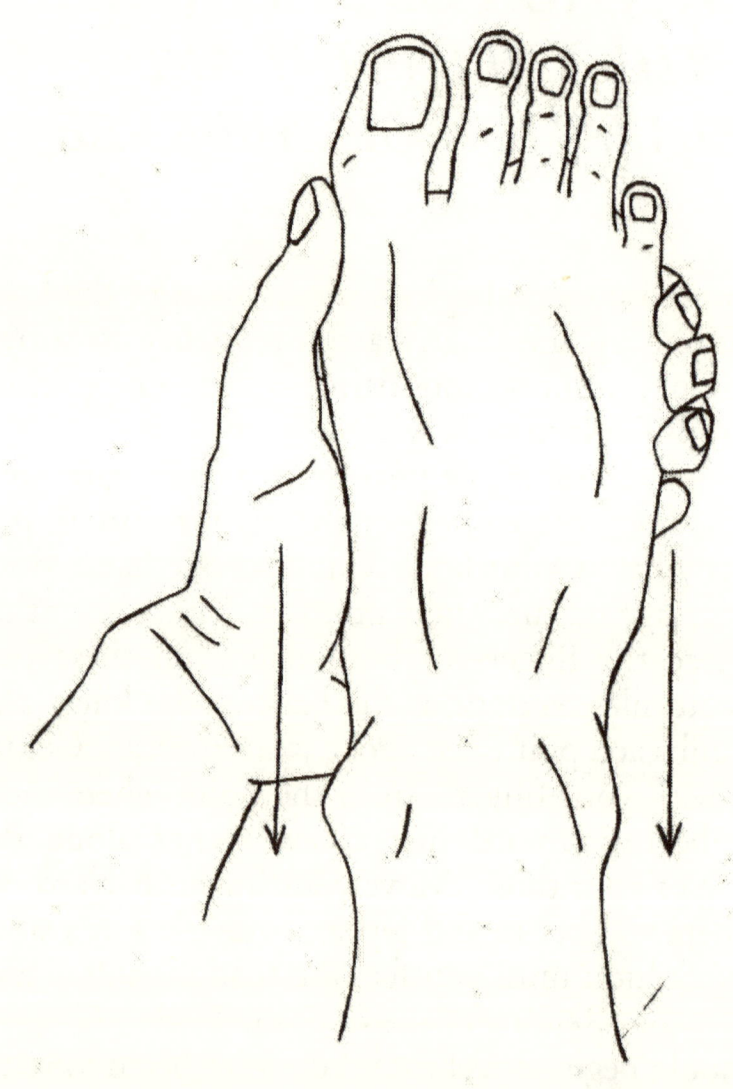

18.
EASING AND PREVENTION OF FOOT PAIN

All of the body weight rests on the feet. Prolonged standing and walking can result in tired and aching feet. Since this can happen on a daily basis, you can massage your feet frequently and if possible, every day. It is recommended to do this exercise either in the morning if you have time, or in the evening after work—before dinner, or two hours after dinner.

Cup your left hand and pour a little massage oil into it. Rub the oil all over the sole of your right foot, including your toes, and around your heel. Gently hold the sides of your right foot with the fingers and thumb of your left hand. Slowly massage the sides of the foot by sliding your fingers and thumb down the sides, from the area just before the toes begin down to the heel. Release, and go back up to the top. Repeat several times.

Now, rub your heel with the fingers of your left hand, in a clockwise fashion, until it begins to feel softer and more relaxed. After this, move to the middle of the sole of your foot and repeat the same clockwise massage here. Then massage the top part of the sole, where the foot meets the toes.

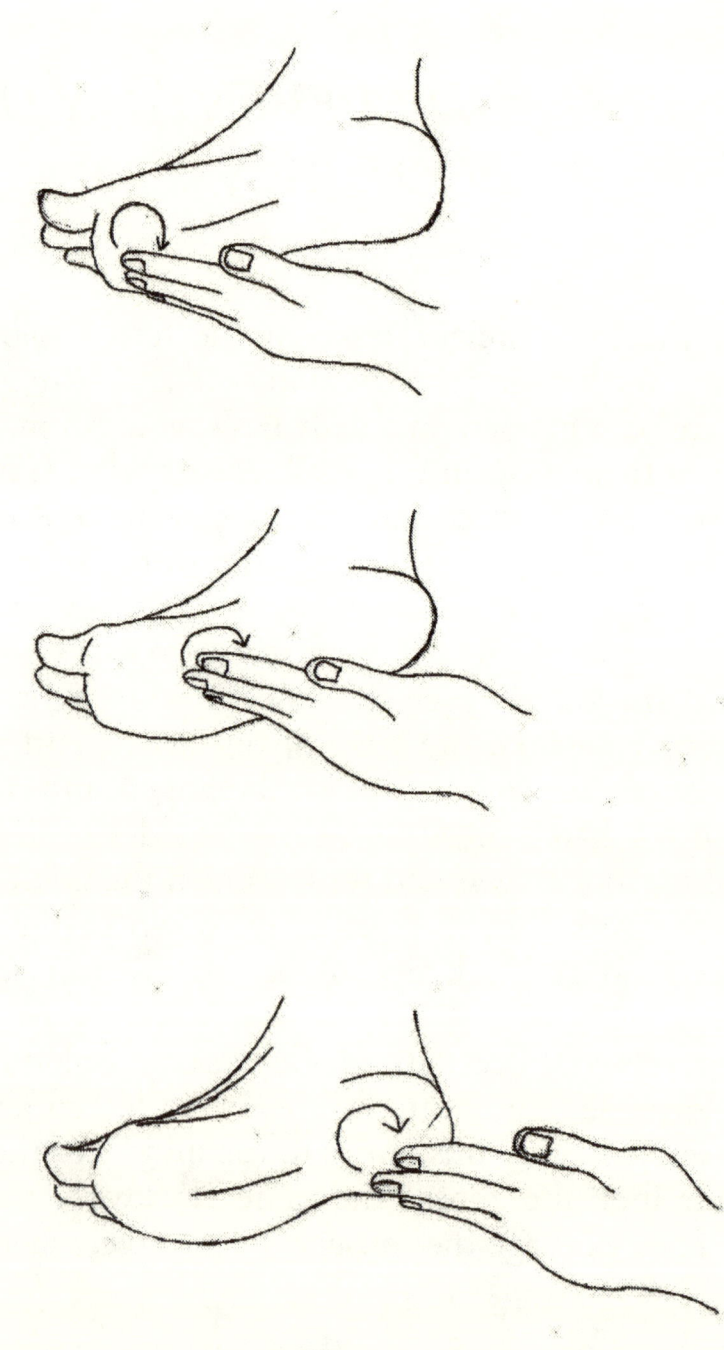

After finishing the entire sole of your foot, rub gently in between the toes with your thumb and fingers, sliding them gently up the sides of each toe. Then take hold of each toe on its sides and press it gently for a few seconds and release.

Repeat this entire massage for your left foot, with your right hand. As your foot warms with the movement of your hand, you can feel it beginning to relax and loosen up. The tension accumulated there is being relieved, and the neurons moving through the various parts of the foot are enlivened as you massage them.

Most of the body's stress accumulates in the feet. The lining in the soles of the feet is made of connective tissue. In order to reduce stress and tension in various parts of the body, daily activation of the connective tissue is highly recommended.

This is also an effective method to stimulate the lymphatic system in your body and help develop the immune system. Most of the lymphatic fluid rests in the sole of your foot and its daily activation keeps you not only relaxed but also healthy.

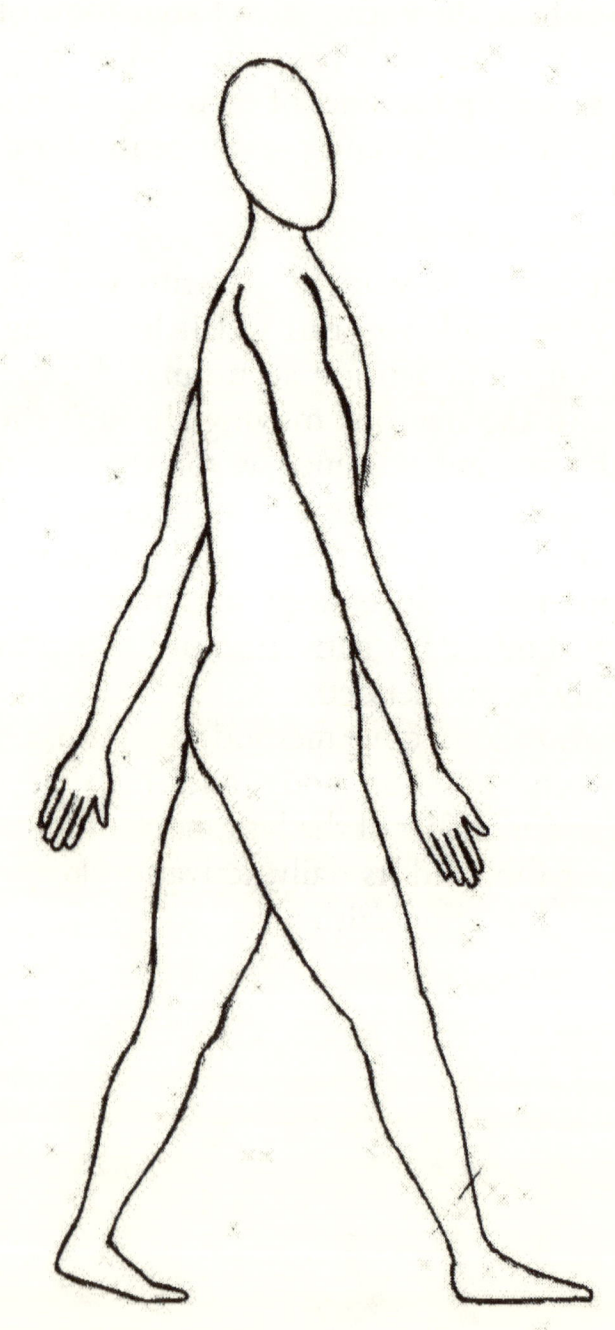

19.
SENSING THE CHI THROUGH
THE ABDOMEN

As you are taking a walk or sitting, pay attention to your abdomen—how it is moving in and out. Now, try to bring this movement in sync with your breath. Breathe in as the abdomen contracts, and breathe out as the abdomen expands. Get into the habit of breathing slowly and rhythmically. Pay attention to the sensations in this area. You may begin to feel subtle energies moving in and through this part of the body. This energy is known in some parts of the Eastern world as "chi," and it is the vital energy of the body.

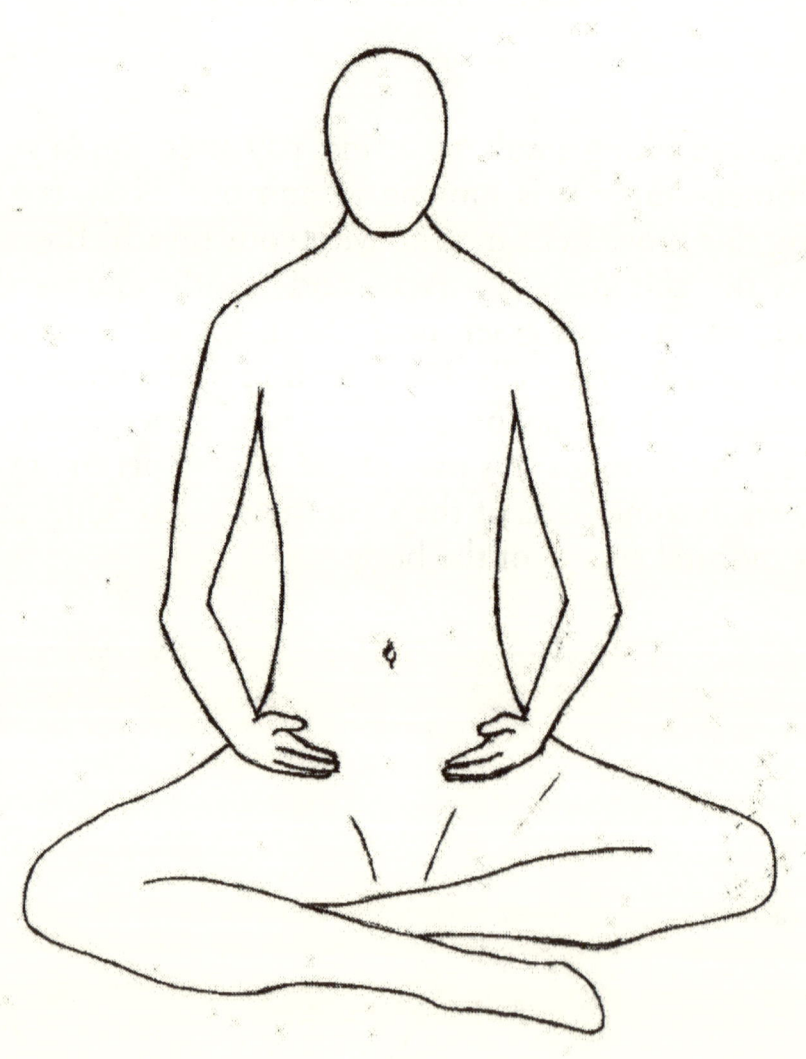

Working with this exercise can also help to flatten and tone your abdominal region. For women and men alike, working with this part of the body can help to avoid the psychological discomfort of not having "the right body." In addition, this exercise can make you more aware of your breath, a helpful tool in becoming more aware of the workings of the entire body.

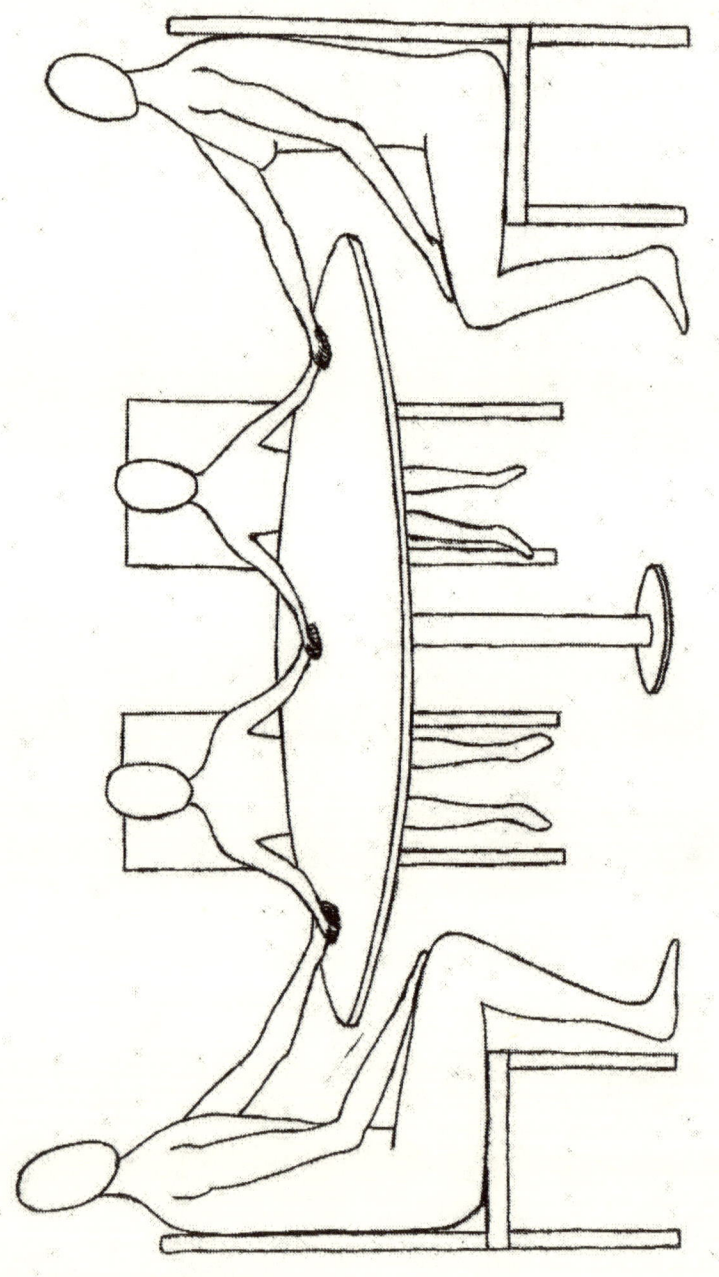

20.
STRESS REDUCTION FOR THE WHOLE FAMILY

This exercise is meant for the entire family. We are not spending enough time together as a family these days. Everyone is involved in something or the other: working, busy with school and homework, attending to unfinished daily chores, etc. It's important to take a few minutes every day together to reinforce each other's sense of being. Although we are separate and individuated, we are also a family unit and this must be acknowledged and celebrated daily.

Before you begin to eat dinner, hold hands around the table. Feel each other. Now breathe together gently—if possible, in unison—and sense a feeling of togetherness, of harmony with each others' presence and vibrations, thus helping to eliminate the scattered and unfocused energies present in each person.

If you are interested, you can enjoy repeating the sound "OM" together for a couple of minutes. This helps to calm down children as well as adults, and helps to keep everyone on the same wavelength.

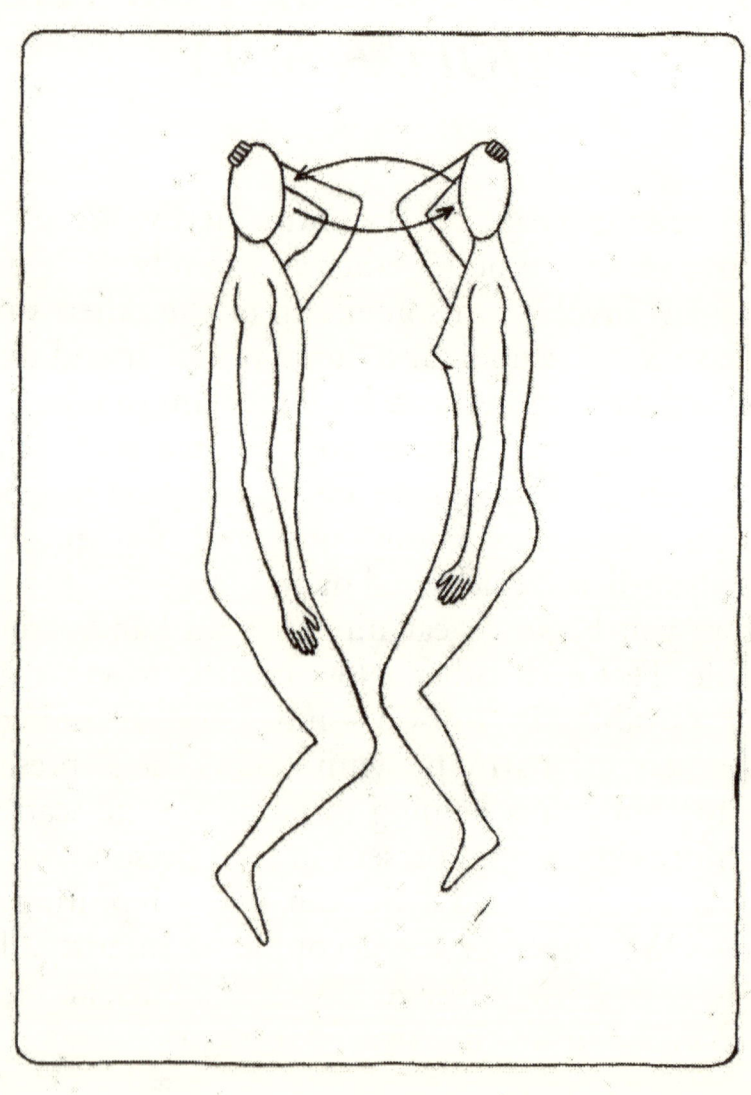

21.
STRESS REDUCTION FOR A MAN AND A WOMAN TOGETHER

With fast-paced and busy lifestyles today, couples are spending less and less time together intimately. Everyone is occupied and not available to their partner. We are eating and drinking more than ever, yet we remain distant and separate from each other's vibrational field. This exercise helps to renew a feeling of intimacy and helps to confirm in us a feeling of togetherness.

Lie down together on a bed, about a foot away from each other. Your eyes should be closed.

For the man: Lie down on your left side, with your left hand resting against your head. This helps the right nostril to open up.

For the woman: Lie down on your right side, with your right hand resting against your head. This helps the left nostril to open up.

As the man breathes out from his right nostril, the woman begins to sense his breath entering her left nostril. As the woman breathes out from her left nostril, the man begins to sense her breath entering his right nostril. No touching is necessary.

What is happening is that you are taking in each other's vital force, with the male energy going into the female, and the female energy going into the male. After a while, an elliptical loop between the two of you begins to form. Repeated used of this ritual leads to relaxation, stress reduction, and a balancing of each other's energy.

THE UNDERSTANDING BEHIND
THE ISOINTEGRAL EXERCISES

Human beings, like the rest of the universe, are made of vibrations. Vibrations have varying wavelengths. Some are short and move rapidly, while others are longer and move more slowly. The various parts of our physical world, though they may seem fixed and inert, are all, upon closer inspection, vibrating. Everything that exists is in movement, in motion, in flux. Everything, from the movements of the planets to elementary particles, is moving in patterns that might best be described as spiral. Within a spiral, there are recognizable cycles, yet these cycles are progressing, evolving, and ever new.

Our own bodies can be seen in the same light. The conglomeration of various types of vibrations comprises the different energetic levels that make up a human being, from the most subtle to the most dense. "Underneath" (this characterization is meant to allude to the finer and more subtle vibrating levels that are intertwined with each other and the physical body, and that build upon each other—the most fine and subtle energies forming the foundation of the whole system) the vibrating physical body lies the vibrating "electrical body." Underneath this "electrical body" lies the unknown "subtle body."

The levels of energy inside us can only be apprehended experientially. Various substances and practices can be (and have been throughout history) used as tools to both experience the levels of one's being, and to consciously work with them.

At a certain point in individual development consciousness, or awareness itself, can be seen as directly interacting with these levels. Perhaps it will even be seen as the "creator" of all of these energetic levels. Our awareness can be used to change, work with, and balance our own internal energies.

The physical illnesses and discomforts so prevalent in American society—among them lower back pain, arthritis, carpal tunnel syndrome, knee joint pain, sleep disorders, and stress—can be directly traced to our lack of awareness of our own internal worlds. The vibrations which constitute the various energies that make up a human being are, in their most dense forms, the very physical tissues, bones, joints, nerves, muscles, and electrical and lymphatic networks that have become hurt or damaged, and which now ail and debilitate us.

Physical pain affects every aspect of our lives, from our strength, energy, and mobility to our thoughts and emotions. These effects extend outward into our lives— into our work, our play, our relationships, even our spirituality.

When we deny the physical (and what lies behind it) through fear or inattention, we cut ourselves off from the roots of our being. For it is through the physical, through our senses, that we may access the subtler levels of energy of which we are made.

If we become interested, and if we decide to take responsibility for our selves, we begin on the path to the reclamation of our true selves. The power is in our hands, so to speak, to fully realize our own inherent power.

At this time, health care costs have become higher than ever, millions are uninsured, and millions have become dependent on medicines that do not address the root causes of our dis-ease.

Realistically, some of our suffering and pain can be alleviated or eliminated without drugs or expensive medical care. Healing can take place from the inside-out, instead of the outside-in, on an ongoing and daily basis.

The path is simple, yet difficult because of the habits and patterns—physical, psychological, and otherwise—that we have developed. Need, desire and interest can lead to attention and increased awareness. Awareness can lead to increased sensitivity. Our senses can be developed and can become attuned to notice the inner workings of our organism. This increased sensitivity can further build upon our awareness. Eventually, we may be able to discern how the various parts and levels within us are interconnected, and how our awareness and our behaviors affect us on a fundamental level. At this point, change and self-healing may be possible.

The IsoIntegral Exercises have been developed to introduce us to our inner worlds through a series of exercises meant to address some of the most commonly occurring conditions and difficulties that people are encountering today. When a disruption or disease manifests in the system, one must entrain oneself through the exercises to become more aware of the existence of the inner bodies.

The ultimate purpose of Yoga and Tibetan Buddhism is to become awakened within oneself. If one is suffering from pain and other bodily discomforts, a certain amount of one's energy is going toward the elimination of that pain and toward feeling fully healthy. That energy is then not available for creating and maintaining the balance and spiritual growth of one's system.

The inner tension that we feel (and even that which we are not yet aware of) leads to an absence of the capacity to enjoy our lives fully. The IsoIntegral Exercises serve to prevent and reduce the pain and suffering in our lives. When we are healthy, both physically and mentally, the exercises may also lay the groundwork for further exploration into the discovery of a higher self that is our birthright.

0-595-30397-8